D0365859

WHEN
Love
HEALS

BY
SAMUEL T. SMITH

with Mary Hutchinson

HIGHERLIFE
PUBLISHING & MARKETING, INC.
Oviedo, Florida

PUBLISHED BY

HigherLife Development Services, Inc.
400 Fontana Circle
Building 1—Suite 105
Oviedo, Florida 32765
(407) 563-4806

www.ahigherlife.com

Printed in the United States

ISBN 13: 978-1-939183-32-3

Unless otherwise indicated, Bible quotations are
taken from the New International Version.[1]

Copywriting and editing: Judi Adamyk,
Mary Frediani, and Melanie Gray with a special
thanks to Beth Filla.

Design and strategy by Inspired Direct, Nashua, NH.
Art Director: Joanne Hemerlein
Production Art: Mary Jane O'Brien
Cover Photo: Greg Bartram
Photography by Medical Ministry International,
with Peru additions by Heidi Hutchinson.

DEDICATION

When Love Heals is dedicated to those people who are in need and do not have a voice. There are 1.4 billion people in developing countries who live on less than $1.25 a day.[1] They need our help. We pray that God will provide a light on the efforts of Medical Ministry International to change their lives.

ACKNOWLEDGEMENTS

The work of Medical Ministry International would not be possible without the passion and support of the MMI Team, Board of Directors, and the over 2,000 volunteers who join with us. The MMI Team thanks our families, supporters, and stewards who provide the love, prayers, and resources that make this ministry work.

I would like to thank God for providing this opportunity to use the skills He has given me. To my wife Jill, thank you for your love, support, and sacrifice to keep our family thriving as your husband spends the many days and weeks away from our home.

Our daughter, Sheridan, and our son, Jensen, you are the lights of our lives and we pray that you too will develop a passion to use the amazing gifts that God has given you to make a difference in the lives of others. Our parents, Ken and Judy Smith and John and Joan Craig, who guided our journey and helped prepare us for this opportunity to serve.

Each one of us has been given amazing gifts of intelligence, resources, and skill. It is my prayer that you will find a way to use these gifts to serve the less fortunate. Jesus provided the guide; it is our calling to use His example to serve others.

Our time on this earth is short, the opportunity to impact lives is now.

"And this is my prayer: that your love may abound more and more in knowledge and depth of insight."

Philippians 1:9

TABLE OF CONTENTS

INTRODUCTION

Let's call her Celia.

Four years old and the youngest of four children, Celia is the apple of her mother's eye. Along with her family, she lives on the bank of a small river deep in the Amazon in what could only be described as a hut, its walls and roof made of grass, sticks, and bamboo.

Celia is a delightful girl with a sweet, contagious laugh. She loves to play, to run, to climb—things that little girls all around the world love to do.

But when her mom called her inside one day, Celia tripped and fell in the dirt. As four-year-olds often do when they get a glimpse of their own blood, she cried. In seconds, her mom was at her side. Gathering Celia in her arms, she hugged her close, kissing away her tears.

Before long, the small cut was forgotten. There was rice to eat for dinner, Daddy would soon be in from the field, and Celia had found a pretty rock to show her mother. All was well.

The next day was the same as the one before, filled with playing and laughter, but by evening, the cut on Celia's knee was starting to bother her. When her mother placed Celia on the bed—nothing more than a straw mat—and told her to go to sleep, Celia fussed and fussed, something she rarely did. By the fourth day, the cut was fiery red and oozing. Celia said it hurt to bend her knee.

LITTLE PROBLEMS LIKE CELIA'S CUT, DIARRHEA, OR CATARACTS BECOME LIFE-THREATENING IN DEVELOPING COUNTRIES.

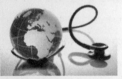

A month later, the little girl's strength was gone; her laughter turned to nothing more than a weak smile. She had a fever her mother could not control. Her leg was on fire and she cried all the time. "What will happen?" her mother silently worried. "Will she lose the use of her leg? Will it cost my child her life?"

This is life in the Amazon, and in many of the places Medical Ministry International serves. The basic medical supplies we take for granted, like an antibiotic cream or a tetanus shot, are virtually unheard of. Things that are little problems to us become life-threatening to them, things like Celia's cut, diarrhea, or cataracts.

In much of the world, medical care is nearly as basic as it was when Jesus walked the earth. In country after country, doctors don't have the training or even the equipment to provide their patients with adequate medical care.

To make matters even scarier, families like Celia's live miles—sometimes hundreds of miles—away from what little medical care is available. Just getting to a hospital is a luxury they simply can't afford; not on the $100 a month this family of six survives on.

I believe you are reading this book for a reason. In the following pages, you will be introduced to 12 people from all over the world who have shared their stories with MMI teams over the past several months.

I have taken some creative liberties to tell their stories in such a way that you will understand the context of their lives, and the challenges faced every day by the world's sick and impoverished. As you read them, their stories will help you see and feel the world through their eyes, their pain, and show you what a difference one gift, one surgery can make.

Each story has taught me a biblical truth that I want to share, giving voice and dialogue to the individuals in the sea of faces we serve.

So please, let me take you along on a journey around the world and show you more. Let me open your eyes to what life is like in developing countries today. Only then can you begin to see those like Celia as our Lord does. It's not enough to simply say, "I love Jesus." We

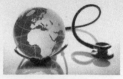

IT'S NOT ENOUGH TO SIMPLY SAY, "I LOVE JESUS." WE MUST PUT THOSE WORDS INTO ACTION.

must put those words into action and help people.

You and I have an opportunity to relieve the suffering of those who cry out from their pain through Medical Ministry International.

Love can still heal, as Jesus did. Let me prove it to you.

> *"Then they cried to the Lord in their trouble,*
> *and he saved them from their distress.*
> *He sent out his word and healed them;*
> *he rescued them from the grave."*
>
> *Psalm 107:19-20*

FAITH FOR RONALD

I am not a doctor. I live in a small town in the US, read my Bible, love coaching little league and watching sports on TV.

In many ways, I am an average American. I have never worried if my children will have enough food to eat, or if the water is safe to drink. I have always known that basic medical issues can be taken care of with a short car ride to a pharmacy or hospital.

But in 2007, my world was changed by a trip to Monrovia, Liberia—a country far outside of my comfort zone. I walked down dusty roads lined with people in need. I met the blind, the lame, the dying. My heart burst with love and compassion for these people who asked for so little, yet needed so much, and I began to see the world through the eyes of Christ.

I learned that God could use the skills He gave me as a marketer and a writer to help these people by giving them a way to tell their stories. As their stories represent not simply words on a page, but real people with real pain that is often easily relieved, I pray you will learn as I did: God wants to use *you* to heal, and through these stories you will see how.

Let's first go to Peru, a beautiful country in South America known for its high mountains and historic ruins. There in the south, near the border of Bolivia, is a city called Arequipa surrounded by three towering mountains. If you look carefully, past

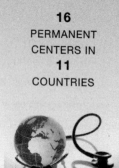

16 PERMANENT CENTERS IN **11** COUNTRIES

the beauty of the snow-capped peaks, you can see thousands and thousands of makeshift huts lining dirt roads in all directions.

For most, the only bathroom is a shallow hole dug in the yard. No privacy, no running water. It costs 35 cents to buy a small bucket of clean water—a huge sum for families that often earn less than $100 a month.

Life is hard, but bearable. That is, until someone is sick. Here is Eva's story, as she struggled to find help for her son:

As told by MMI physical therapist, Jodee

"Help me walk, Mama, help me walk."

Those words hurt my heart every time I hear Ronald beg his mom, Eva.

Ronald was born premature at only seven months. Because of his low birth weight and lack of oxygen during Eva's pregnancy, he spent his first 21 days fighting for his life in an incubator at the hospital. Thankfully, Ronald made it through those rough early days.

When he finally went home, Eva thought the worst was over; she had no reason to think there was anything else wrong with him.

But from the time he was one year old, Eva started to notice that something wasn't right. His struggle to walk was beyond that of a normal toddler and no matter how hard he tried, his walking did not improve. Weeks went by and finally Eva brought him to the local hospital. The doctor didn't seem worried, and suggested she take him to a government clinic for therapy.

Eva wanted to be hopeful that this would help, but she knew better than to get her hopes up; the first few years of a child's life are critical for development, and Ronald was already far behind. His mother loved him so much but she was fearful for how this might affect his future.

Eva explained to me one day, "Life for our family is hard enough and I don't want Ronald to struggle even more. My husband works hard every day, trying to do what he can so that I can take care of Ronald. We have food, but nothing extra."

When she took him to a local therapist, Eva learned that Ronald had cerebral palsy (CP) caused by a lack of oxygen before birth. CP is a general term and it means different things for different kids.

For Ronald, it meant he couldn't move the lower half of his body—a condition called "diplegia." He used his arms pretty normally, but he didn't have much strength in his legs, and his feet were turned inward. Both of those things made walking very, very difficult.

The therapist at the hospital told her about Medical Ministry International. Her words gave Eva her first real hope. The local doctors had no way to help him, and she was so desperate it didn't matter that our clinic was a five-hour bus ride away.

Once they had signed in, I led them to the examination room and laid Ronald on the bed in front of me. I could tell Eva was nervous, so I started talking with her to calm her down, asking her questions about Ronald's medical history as I tested his legs and other muscles.

I explained that Ronald would need therapy at the clinic every week. He would need braces—braces we could give him—that would build his muscle strength, and one day he would walk.

While this is good news for Eva and Ronald, I know it is still hard on their entire family. Eva tells me, "My husband sacrifices so that we only make the trip once a week. Ronald and I stay in a rooming house for three days while he goes to physical therapy. Then we make the journey back home for the other four days."

But despite the struggle, Eva is determined, "Yes, it puts stress on my family, but the gift of my child walking is worth everything my family does. I have faith in Ronald; he is so determined. And I have faith in MMI.

"When he started therapy, Ronald couldn't walk or even talk. Now, he can talk like any other three-year-old. He crawls, and can raise himself up to walk, and I know he would not have made this kind of progress at the local hospital."

Ronald and Eva work hard at this, doing the exercises each day they are not at MMI's clinic. He, too, has hope and tells her, "I really want to walk. I want to run."

OVER 250 VOLUNTEERS SENT TO PERU ANNUALLY

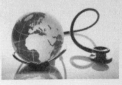

Even if Ronald never walks on his own, he would not have made the progress he *has made without MMI's help. We have given Ronald a chance at a better life.*

Jesus told His disciples to, "Come, follow me" (Mark 1:17). Faith in Jesus Christ is not a passive faith; it is an active faith, a doing faith. Nothing says "Jesus loves you" to Ronald's mother more than MMI helping her child walk.

The miracle of this child walking is a credit to the physical therapists who work with him each week, the teams of doctors, nurses, and volunteers who come every few months, and the faithful donors who give to make it all possible. We each play our role; we each share the burden and the reward.

Ronald walks. Jesus smiles. And everyone who touches this child is blessed.

"Great crowds came to him, bringing the lame, the blind, the crippled, the mute and many others, and laid them at his feet; and he healed them. The people were amazed when they saw the mute speaking, the crippled made well, the lame walking and the blind seeing. And they praised the God of Israel."

Matthew 15:30-31

WHERE LOVE TOOK ANTONIO

Because of its history, Colombia may not immediately conjure up images of God's love. The drug cartels have been the focus of headlines for so long; it is too easy to forget the people there, the good, hardworking people who struggle against poverty every single day.

God loves these dear people as much as He loves you and me. His grace is manifested in many ways, not the least of which is through MMI.

Through every surgery, every life changed, we are showing the meaning of 1 Corinthians 13:13, "And now these three remain: faith, hope and love. But the greatest of these is love." The greatest force in the world is love.

The following is a love story that touches my heart, and expresses both the love of God and the love of a woman for her husband. Below, we see Antonio, a man who suffered from blindness, through his wife's eyes:

Three years ago, my husband started to lose his eyesight.

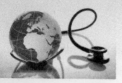

$500
GIVES
SIGHT TO
THE BLIND

At 56, his vision became blurry, making it difficult to see, until it was completely gone. In our country of Colombia, people are either very rich or they are very poor. Life for us wasn't impossible, but with my husband's vision gone, only I could work, and it became an absolute burden to provide for our family.

I saw how hard life became for Antonio after that. On top of having to adjust to life without sight, he was no longer able to take care of his family, and I knew how that broke his heart.

For two years, we lived like that. Him, coping with the loss of his sight. Me, coping with the doubled work load, taking care of him and our family. I knew we could not live like this for much longer; I was getting too old to do all the work by myself, and I missed the happy, cheerful man my husband used to be.

Our insurance company wanted him to go to Bogotá for surgery, but he didn't want to. He had heard about Medical Ministry International, and he had his heart set on going there. He told me, "Something beautiful is happening at the MMI clinic, and I trust the doctors there more than any in Bogotá."

I hadn't seen my husband so determined, so passionate about something since he lost his eyesight; some of his old self was coming back. I wasn't about to lose that, so I promised him we would do whatever it took for us to get in to their clinic.

We went to visit the MMI clinic and found that they could not book his surgery that year; there were too many patients and not enough time for everyone.

My husband was disappointed, but he would not be seen anywhere else. He put his name on the list for the following year when they could guarantee him the right amount of time for surgery and recovery.

So one year later, days after his 59th birthday, my husband and I returned to the MMI clinic. I wasn't allowed with him in the preparation room, during the surgery, or after in the recovery room.

He must have been so lonely, and maybe even scared. My husband is a strong man, but he wanted so badly for the surgery to work; we both did. After, he told me that all the doctors and nurses were so kind to him; they made him feel comfortable.

When he walked out of the recovery room, our eyes locked for the first time in three years. I began to weep.

The surgery had worked!

Antonio kept repeating, "It is the best birthday gift I could have ever received." He is so grateful to MMI; we both are. They gave us so much more than just Antonio's sight. They gave my husband back to me, and they gave his livelihood, his happiness back to him. He is a new man, now, thanks to MMI.

23
COUNTRIES
SERVED IN 2012

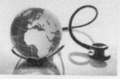

Love is the very basis of everything we do at MMI. We are the hands and feet of the Lord (1 Corinthians 12) who loved us enough to die for us, and we hope to share some of that love with everyone we touch, including Antonio and his wife.

The Lord asks today that we hear the cry of the poor, the weak, the blind. What better way to show it than love them with the love He gave us?

> *"If I give all I possess to the poor and give over my body to hardship that I may boast, but do not have love, I gain nothing."*

> ***1 Corinthians 13:3***

BERISSO WAITS FOR GOD

As a Baby Boomer, the drought in Ethiopia that started in 1970[1] was my first introduction to dire poverty. Over 1.2 million people died.[2] Like every church attendee of the day, I saw the slideshows of frail children on the brink of death, bellies bloated, flies crawling across listless faces.

Today in Ethiopia, clean water is scarce and the average life span is less than 60 years.[3] It is estimated that there are only 103 ophthalmologists with surgical skills for the near 83 million people.[4]

In the midst of such a grave situation, MMI is an oasis of hope, offering life-changing medical care. We are blessed to know the story of Berisso, an inspirational man in Meki, Ethiopia. Let Berisso's son tell his story:

My dad is the strongest man I know.

He's a great dad to my 10 siblings and me. Even though some of us don't live at home anymore, at one time or another, we have all depended on him for everything—food, money, advice, love.

For as long as I can remember, my dad has needed a wheelchair. The dirt roads that lead through our village weren't made for wheelchairs. Dodging potholes and rocks is too much for him so he can't make any trip alone; one of us needs to push him up the hills and pull him out when he gets stuck in a hole.

It might be easier to see my dad live with his disability if the other villagers weren't so mean to him. No one makes eye contact with him when he passes; no one comes to help him if he gets stuck. Here in Ethiopia, any disability is considered a curse from God and so no one will associate with my dad.

But he meets their ridicule with kindness, telling me not to be angry with God or my neighbors, refusing to believe his disability is a curse. He tells me it is the way God made him, and that's enough for my dad. Yes, he gets frustrated by the things he can't do, but he relies on God for strength in those times.

Knowing how strong my dad is, I never really worried about him. But a few years ago, he started losing his vision. It happened slowly, like the light fading away at dusk. He knew total darkness was coming, but he had to wait a long time before he could go to a hospital.

Life got so much harder for him. Soon he wasn't able to see the bumps in the road anymore as he struggled with his wheelchair; when he was alone he couldn't do anything to prevent himself from running into someone or something.

Sure, he had us kids to take him places and help him around the house, but unless we all worked and sold the food from our small farm, there would be no money, so we couldn't be home all day.

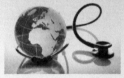

$200
WILL PAY
FOR A
REFURBISHED
WHEELCHAIR

When we finally saved up enough money for the surgery, it was the happiest I had seen him in years. He was going to see again; his life was about to become much easier.

I went with him to the government hospital. It took us hours to get to there, and when we finally made it, we received terrible news, "You only have enough money for one surgery, on one eye."

My dad's face fell. But there was still a small glimmer of hope in his eyes. He agreed to the one surgery and they rolled him away for preparation.

The surgery was a success, and my dad was able to see out of one of his eyes again. He had become so used to not having any sight that now, with sight in one eye, he was a new man.

He could move around the house again and even around a few areas of the neighborhood. And he was determined more than ever to get surgery for his second eye.

All of that—the first surgery and the decision to save for the second surgery—happened seven years ago. My dad still didn't have the money for the surgery, and cataracts began to re-form in his first eye, causing his vision to deteriorate once again.

It was so hard for him to find value, to find worth. Now the village mocked him and avoided him even more than before; it was like he didn't exist. He couldn't go anywhere without help from someone—not to bed, not to the bathroom, not to the garden to get food for himself.

One day when Dad was really discouraged, I decided to go for a walk with him. While we were out in the village, we heard an announcement that there was a Medical Ministry International eye clinic coming nearby in one week.

My dad was so excited. He had heard good things about MMI and he told me, "They are doing God's work, and I know they will be able to help me."

The moment we went back to the hut he started counting down the days. Every morning when he woke up he would tell me, "Six days" or "Five days" right down until the morning when he told me, "Today is the day!"

We made our way to the clinic and the minute we walked through the doors, I could tell my dad was at peace. All the nurses and doctors were so kind to him. It was obvious they truly cared, so I wasn't worried when they took him to be prepared for surgery.

The surgery went well and now my dad can see again—in both eyes! He is so grateful to God and to MMI. They have given my father the greatest gift he could ever receive, and they did it in the name of God. MMI has changed my father's entire life.

2,710
PATIENTS
SERVED IN
ETHIOPIA
IN 2012

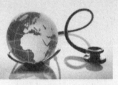

Everything Jesus did was intended to share God's love with all who would come and listen. Jesus did not just teach through words, but also through actions.

He healed the sick out of compassion for their struggles. He sought to help people, explaining how serving the less fortunate was actually serving God. Jesus was the supreme example of His own teaching.

Even as far away as Ethiopia is, it is not so distant

that you can't offer a healing hand. A surgery like the one Berisso needed costs only $500. It changes lives! It helps entire families. It witnesses to the whole village.

"Heal the sick, raise the dead, cleanse those who have leprosy, drive out demons. Freely you have received; freely give."

Matthew 10:8

NEW LIFE FOR ISAC

In Mark 5, starting at verse 40, we find a story that is chilling to every parent who reads it. A little girl was dying and there was nothing her parents could do—nothing but ask Jesus for a miracle:

"After he put them all out, he took the child's father and mother and the disciples who were with him, and went in where the child was. He took her by the hand and said to her, *'Talitha koum!'* (which means 'Little girl, I say to you, get up!'). Immediately the girl stood up and began to walk around (she was twelve years old). At this they were completely astonished."

All over the region, people talked about the great love that Jesus showed, healing people, spending time with them, sharing from His heart as He traveled. He had the power, He had the heart; the only thing the girl needed was His attention for a moment.

But the story of this little girl ends strangely: Jesus didn't want her parents to tell (Mark 5:43). How could they not tell? It must have been the most difficult secret they kept their entire lives!

Our ministry met Diego, a man from Peru who faced a similar tragedy. His son was dying. In fact, Diego thought he was dead. But he'll never be able to keep it a secret. Let him tell the story:

Just six weeks ago, my wife Mariana gave birth to a beautiful baby boy. As I held little Isac, I knew what it felt like for a dream to come true.

Mariana and I wanted a baby for a long time, but we weren't sure we'd ever be able to provide for one. We had a hard enough time feeding ourselves that we couldn't guarantee we'd be able to keep a baby alive, too.

When I found out Mariana was pregnant, I put all my efforts into the business I was trying to start. I have a small stand at the village market. Perhaps it doesn't seem like much, just long hours standing in the sun behind a wooden table on one of the side roads, but I like the people I meet and I have great pride in my work.

Every day I go to the market with a smile on my face and hope in my heart that this will be the day, that today I will have enough customers to expand my business. Then I could have two tables, offer more things to my customers, and really support my family.

When my son was born I was so excited. Mariana

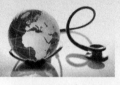

24/7
ACCESS
TO CARE
AT MMI CLÍNICA
LETICIA

and Isac were able to come home two days later, both healthy and happy. As I took them home, I thought, "I'm the luckiest man alive."

But it soon became a nightmare. About a month after Isac was born, I woke up one morning and looked for a few pieces of bread to eat for breakfast before going to work. Our house is very small, just two little rooms. One we sleep in, and the other has a small table, two chairs, and some mats on the floor.

From our bedroom just a few feet away, I heard a shriek. My heart racing, I rushed to Mariana's side. She was in the room holding Isac, her ear on the tiny chest. And then she sobbed, "He's…not…breathing!"

We tried rubbing his chest, doing anything we could think to try. Nothing happened. Finally all hope was gone. We wept until there were no more tears.

Later that day, we had the sad job of looking for a coffin for our one-month-old baby boy. I didn't know they made coffins that small; no parent should ever need one. My wife came with me, carrying our lifeless bundle in her arms.

As I waited to pay, an older woman looked at me strangely. "What are you doing?" she asked.

I was mad to hear her words. Couldn't she see what we were doing? We were buying the one thing a parent never wants to buy for their child: a coffin. "We're looking for a coffin for our baby," I said loudly, angry to even have to respond.

But the woman grabbed my arm and responded, "But your baby is breathing!"

My heart stopped. Could it be? Could Isac be alive? My wife quickly checked and sure enough our baby was breathing the tiniest, shortest breaths!

It was a miracle he was alive, but we had to get help. I didn't know what was wrong, but I knew he needed a doctor. We worked quickly to find a picka picka (a small, motorized dug-out canoe) and made our way to a place I knew could help my baby: Medical Ministry International Clínica Leticia, a four-hour journey down the Amazon River.

The boat moved quickly, but it didn't seem fast enough for me. At long last I could see the village around the curve of the river. As soon as we grounded the canoe, I picked up Isac and started running. I ran as fast as I could until I made it to the clinic, screaming for someone to help my son.

Their emergency pediatric response team rushed out to meet me, and as I handed Isac to them, I was overwhelmed with a sense of calm. I just knew they would be able to save him.

After four days, my son was still hooked up to all sorts of machines, but the doctors told my wife and me that he would live!

47
EMERGENCY ROOM
PATIENTS TREATED
EACH DAY AT
MMI CLÍNICA LETICIA

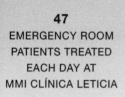

Today my family is back home again and almost everything is back to normal; only my morning routine has changed. When I wake up now, the first things I do are kiss my wife and son. MMI saved the most important thing in the world to me: my family.

Without MMI, would Isac's story have ended the same way? I doubt it. The first-class medical intervention that saved this baby boy was unlike anything any other clinic in the Amazon could have done.

Is Diego's child less important than your child or grandchild, than the little girl in biblical days? Jesus doesn't think so. It was His love, through our doctors and nurses, that brought Isac back from death's door.

What a story, what a Savior!

"And the prayer offered in faith
will make the sick person well;
the Lord will raise them up.
If they have sinned, they will be forgiven."

James 5:15

FOLLOWING SOFÍA'S STEP

> "I pledge allegiance to the Lamb, with all my
> strength, with all I am. I will seek to follow His
> commands. I pledge allegiance to the Lamb."

"I Pledge Allegiance to the Lamb" by Ray Boltz is one of my all-time favorite songs, as the lyrics are so powerful. Following God's commands with my all is my daily assignment.

And following doesn't come easy for me. I am a leader, a doer, but I have learned that good things truly happen to those who wait, who show the Lord that they trust His timing more than their own human understanding. When I place my footsteps in His, amazing things happen.

Maybe this is why I was so touched by the following story about a man who had no other option but to physically follow his wife. Let it bless you:

As told by MMI doctor, Joe Fammartino

I remember the couple very well. It was a few years ago. Our 12-hour surgery schedule was more than full. Pausing for a moment between operations, I looked up the street to see a woman leading a man down the dusty street towards the medical clinic in Barranquilla, Colombia.

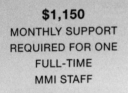

$1,150
MONTHLY SUPPORT
REQUIRED FOR ONE
FULL-TIME
MMI STAFF

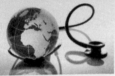

Motorbikes, starving dogs and ancient cars all gave them a wide berth as they slowly made their way towards us. The woman's face captured my attention at once. I had no idea how old she was, but the lines on her face and the set of her jaw spoke of pain, hard work, and little hope.

Behind, her husband had one hand on her shoulder; the other carried a small, worn bag. They walked slowly, wordlessly, edging towards us with each step.

Their tattered clothes told their story for them. No doubt the husband had worked every day on a local farm, bringing in most of the money, as little as it might have been.

And now, because the man could no longer see, he was unable to work. I can only imagine what a burden this must have been on his wife, knowing that it was up to her to provide for their family.

I left my spot by the window and took a seat in the examination room, a simple 8' by 8' room, smaller than most of my closets back in the States. Everything around me was medically adequate but sparse; as an ophthalmologist, I had the bare minimum of what I needed, which was sadly much more than the doctors in Barranquilla had before we arrived.

After the couple signed in and registered, they introduced themselves as Santiago and Sofia. I managed to do a quick exam to see if we could help him. The diagnosis made me both angry and glad at the same time: the man had bilateral cataracts.

In the United States, this surgery would be easy to have done in a day. It is so simple, yet in this country, it was out of reach to most of the population. Until Medical Ministry International started working in Colombia, having cataracts meant a life sentence of blindness for most people. But for Santiago, we could give him back his sight!

The need for surgery is so great in Colombia that our schedules fill up quickly, and this trip was no different. Our time in the country was almost through, so we would only be able to perform surgery on one eye.

I gently explained that we would fix one eye that day. If he would come back the next year, we would fix the other eye.

Neither of them reacted to my words. I'm not sure they knew how to hope anymore. Thankfully, the first surgery went perfectly.

Hours later, as Santiago peered out the one good eye in recovery, his entire demeanor seemed to change. He was happier, he seemed stronger, and the love in the look he and his wife exchanged brought me to tears. Before leaving, Santiago promised to try to come back the next year.

One year later, back on the ground in Barranquilla, I found myself constantly on the lookout for Santiago and Sofía. Sure enough, on our second day there, they came back, eager for us to fix his other eye.

The second surgery went just as perfectly as the first, and he was a changed man.

I did not expect to see the couple again. I never left the medical base while I was in country and since the surgeries had restored his eyesight; there was no reason for him to return.

Still, I thought of them often and wondered how their lives had changed. On my third trip to Barranquilla, a year after I had operated on Santiago's second eye, we were on the bus from the airport to the clinic when I saw a man I thought I recognized in the distance ahead.

Roads in Colombia are never empty, so I was able to get a good look at him while we crawled through the busy traffic. We made eye contact and his mouth turned into a beaming smile. It was Santiago!

Santiago ran towards me, shoved his entire upper body through the bus window and gave me the biggest hug! Through his excitement, he pointed back to the kiosk I had seen him near as he told me that was his; he owned it. Now that he was able to see, he had his own business and

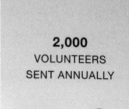

2,000
VOLUNTEERS
SENT ANNUALLY

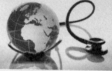

was able to provide for his family again!

My wife and I always say that people universally smile in the same language. I didn't speak Santiago's language, but I spoke his joy and I shared it with him.

Following Christ is never the easy road. He told the rich young ruler to sell everything he owned to follow Him (Mark 10). He asked His disciples to leave their businesses, their mothers and fathers, everything they knew to follow Him (Luke 5).

What is God asking you to do today to follow

Him? Is He bidding you to come with us and use your talent—be it hospitality, teaching, photography or childcare—to minister to people halfway around the world?

Or, is He bidding you to allow someone else to go and serve with your gift, giving up something that matters to you so that you can give a life-changing surgery to someone you will never meet, but who is close to His heart?

Follow Him. His footsteps. His plan.

> *"Trust in the Lord with all your heart*
> *and lean not on your own understanding;*
> *in all your ways submit to him,*
> *and he will make your paths straight."*
>
> *Proverbs 3:5-6*

ESTHER'S LOVE

Jesus spent a lot of time with women who were outcasts of society.

To the woman caught in adultery, His words shamed an angry crowd, sparing her life, challenging her to go and sin no more (John 8). To the woman at the well with a list of prior husbands and another man living with her, He offered her Living Water (John 4).

Our doctors and nurses are often given the opportunity to show Christ's love to people whose sins have devastated their lives, to people whose sins have made them outcasts.

Beyond meeting the obvious physical needs, our job is to show compassion and grace.

Let me introduce you to Esther, a woman in Ghana whose heart was surely broken, whose choices left her not only struggling daily to survive as a single woman on her own, but with a child she originally didn't want.

You can feel her pain in her story:

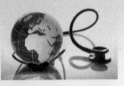

47,423
PATIENTS
SERVED IN
GHANA IN 2012

My boyfriend told me he loved me and that he wanted to be with me forever, and I believed him.

But he changed his mind when I became pregnant. He told me he didn't want anything to do with me, that it wasn't "his problem" because we were not married.

I begged him to stay, hoping he would want to marry me someday, but he refused. He left me as soon as my pregnancy became obvious.

My next decision seemed easy: I was going to get rid of the baby. But the options were all painful. I considered having an abortion, but I couldn't bring myself to do it, so I decided I would give birth to the baby and then leave it somewhere.

Not far from where I live, there is a dump where people come and go all the time. If I left the baby there, someone would find it quickly and make sure everything was okay. That sounded like the best idea; keeping the baby was never an option.

In Ghana, single mothers are looked at with scorn. It is a shameful thing to have a baby and no husband, and

I knew if I kept the baby I would never be able to find a husband in the future. I would never be able to have the family I want to have; my life would be over. I told myself over and over that getting rid of the baby was the best choice for me.

The pregnancy was so hard. People talked about me, would not look me in the eye once I was showing. I was all alone. My family would have nothing to do with me, and no one would help.

When the baby was almost ready to be born, I heard about Medical Ministry International on the radio. I didn't know where else to go to have the baby; I was afraid someone at the government hospital might recognize me and make me feel terrible, so I decided to go to the MMI clinic.

I decided after I gave birth, when the nurses took the baby out of the delivery room, I would sneak out and leave it with them. This seemed like a good plan. After all, it was a baby clinic—they would have the right things to take care of the baby; I didn't know how to take care of it by myself.

So I had the baby and everything went fine. I had every intention of leaving once the medical team was out of the room, but I was too exhausted and I fell asleep.

A short while later, I woke up to see a nurse with a

gentle face holding my baby in the chair next to my bed. She was talking softly to the baby, I suppose so she would not wake me. When I sat up she stood and started to hand me the baby.

"No!" I said.

She looked confused, almost hurt.

"No," I said again. "I don't want it," shaking my head.

I tried to get up but the nurse stopped me, asked me to wait a moment, and then left. Just when I was about to finally leave, she came back with food for the baby and me.

I was so hungry. I couldn't remember how long it had been since I had eaten. As I ate my meal, I saw how affectionate the nurse was to the baby. For a moment, I felt a small pang in my heart and it felt good; I was starting to love my child. I asked to hold the baby and she smiled a big smile, and handed my baby to me.

The moment I felt the small body in my arms, I knew I would never be able to let go again. I loved this baby; I wanted to be a mother to this baby.

I spent the next week there, taking care of my baby and myself so that we would be healthy to begin our new life together once we left the clinic. All the nurses watched me hesitantly. I know they all thought I would leave the baby in the clinic. But I was never going to

above

Ronald playing with physical therapist Jodee, who believes that physical therapy should be as fun as it is beneficial.

below

Berisso waiting for the surgery that will give him sight for the first time in six years.

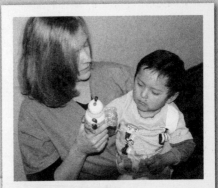

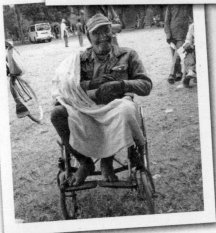

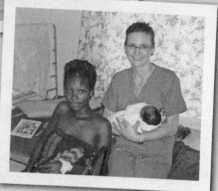

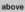
above
Isac tucked in
bed, recovering
in MMI Clínica
Leticia's
24-hour
emergency
clinic.

below
After seeing the love of MMI's staff,
Esther decided to keep her baby.

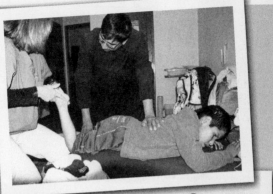

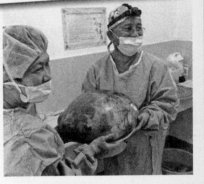

above
Because of MMI's help, the priest's compassion, and Jimmy's hard work, Jimmy will walk!

below
MMI surgeons holding Lin's 46-pound tumor.

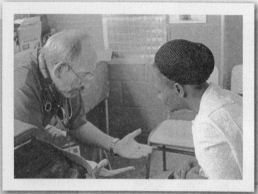

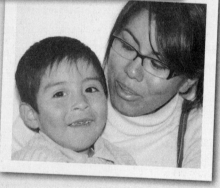

above

Dr. Henry Bush, a doctor who serves with MMI, praying for Fabiola's health and healing after her visit to the MMI clinic.

below

Didier in the arms of his dedicated mother.

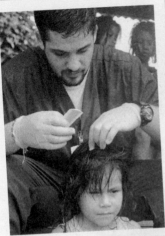

above
Chance delousing one of the children in Colombia.

below
Chance and the MMI Team traveling down the Amazon in a banana boat.

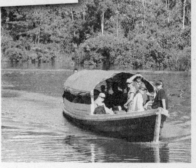

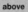

above

Dr. Joe Fammartino checking on a patient in Boca Chica, Dominican Republic.

Photo courtesy of Elizabeth Opalenik and Rita Villanueva.

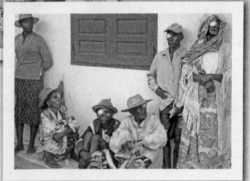

below

Patients recovering from eye surgery in Malawi.

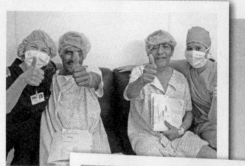

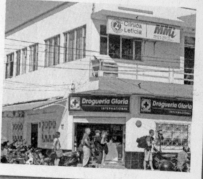

above
Ready to go!
Patients give
their surgeons
the thumbs
up for surgery
in Tabasco,
Mexico.

below
MMI Clínica Leticia headquarters in the Amazon
Region of Colombia.

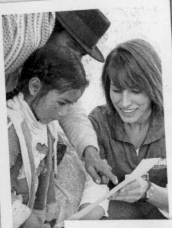

above
MMI volunteer communicating across language barriers in Ayacucho, Peru.

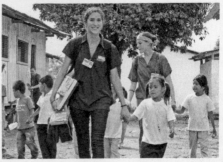

below
MMI volunteers working with children so they can have a healthy future.

leave my baby.

Later, my child and I left the MMI clinic ready for our new life together. I thanked the nurses, hugged them, and went on my way. I am so thankful for the kindness and affection the MMI nurses showed us.

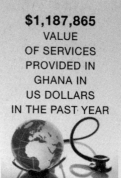

$1,187,865
VALUE
OF SERVICES
PROVIDED IN
GHANA IN
US DOLLARS
IN THE PAST YEAR

They were more than just doctors and nurses; they showed me love.

Love is a powerful force. It's so powerful that Esther could not ignore the feeling of love when the nurses were holding her baby. She probably hadn't felt love in a long time. Her boyfriend left her, her family wouldn't talk to her, and no one in her community wanted to be around her.

She was a stranger to love, so how could she be expected to love her own child?

But then she saw the little bundle in the nurse's arms, and that was all it took. At MMI, our job is more than meeting the physical needs of our patients. We minister with love and compassion so all our patients know they have value to God and to us.

Esther couldn't go anywhere else for help; everyone

had turned her away. But at our clinic, we welcome women like her; we are there for them, showing them what it means to really love.

*"By this everyone will know that you
are my disciples,
if you love one another."*

John 13:35

GOD DIDN'T ORPHAN JIMMY

The concept of abandoning your child at an orphanage is difficult for most Americans to understand. I don't understand it, but I see it all the time in the countries I visit.

The term "economic orphans" applies to many of the orphans in these institutions, meaning their parents decide they can no longer afford to care for them. Perhaps they have too many children, so they keep some and give up others so they don't all starve to death.

Sometimes there is no work and the parents decide to leave the country, hoping to find a job and perhaps reunite with their children later.

In Jimmy's case, he was abandoned at a Catholic orphanage in Peru because he was badly hurt in a fall. His medical situation must have seemed too overwhelming; he couldn't be left alone for one moment.

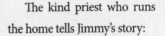

45
YEARS MMI
HAS BEEN
MINISTERING
TO THE POOR

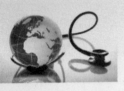

The kind priest who runs the home tells Jimmy's story:

When I look at Jimmy, my heart breaks.

Although his head is covered in thick black hair, you can still see the jagged scars running across his scalp. His head must have shattered like a cracked egg. Like Humpty Dumpty in the childhood story, the doctors were unable to put Jimmy back together the way he was before. His body is twisted and his eyes are glazed over from medication for his brain damage.

But Jimmy was not always this way. He was a healthy, happy eight-year-old boy with a bright future before him. He lived with his mother and father until tragedy changed his life forever: he somehow fell two stories headfirst onto a tile floor.

It has been three years since his fall. Now, at the age of 11, Jimmy isn't able to speak more than a few words. He walks on his tiptoes because his muscles are so tight that he can't relax them to walk on the bottoms of his feet, and he sucks his thumb like a two-year-old.

Jimmy's parents put him in our orphanage for special

needs children. Our hearts are big, but our money is small. Specialized care for a child like Jimmy is very expensive and hard to find—that is, besides at Medical Ministry International's clinic.

It is a long journey filled with bus rides and bumpy roads, but Jimmy and I continue to make it to the MMI clinic. They were the first people to give me good news about Jimmy: one day he will walk!

Since our first visit, we have been getting him used to a brace that allows his muscles to relax so he can walk on the bottoms of his feet. I can tell he's uncomfortable, but I know it will help him in the future.

Even though his muscles are still very tight, I am told if I work with him the way the MMI team is teaching me, and if I bring him to the clinic every week, he will walk.

Without MMI, I know I would never have been able to help Jimmy in this way. No one cared about this helpless

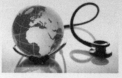

$8
VALUE OF EVERY
$1 GIVEN TO
MMI FOR
MEDICAL SERVICES

child until we came to MMI's clinic. No matter what I have to do, no matter how far I need to travel, I will do it for Jimmy. MMI is an answer to prayer.

From just this one home, MMI sees three orphans for weekly medical care. With barely enough money to pay for basic necessities like food and water, the specialized care that Jimmy needs is more than they could afford.

But we as Christians have a special obligation to the orphans. James 1:27 says, "Religion that God our Father accepts as pure and faultless is this: to look after orphans and widows in their distress and to keep oneself from being polluted by the world."

Today there are more than 130 million orphans in the world—almost half the population of the United States![1] They are street children, trafficked children, soldier children; the lucky ones are in loving homes like the one Jimmy is in.

One day each of us will stand before the Lord and He will ask this question: "What did you do with the gifts I gave you to help my orphans?" I want to have a good answer, don't you?

"I will not leave you as orphans;
I will come to you."

John 14:18

AN ANSWER FOR MARÍA

The things that grow in the Amazon amaze me. There are flowers so stunning they take my breath away, strange trees unlike anything I have ever seen, bushes and vines of every description. There are at least 40,000 different plant species in Colombia alone; that's 10% of the world's plant species in one country![1]

What a creative God we serve!

In John 15, Jesus uses plants as metaphors for the importance of His Word in our lives, "I am the true vine, and my Father is the gardener. He cuts off every branch in me that bears no fruit, while every branch that does bear fruit he prunes so that it will be even more fruitful" (1-2). We get our nourishment in His Spirit which allows us to grow, to learn and to please Him.

Nothing is more important in our Christian walk than the Word of God, which is why I was thrilled when I heard why María wanted her sight improved:

I didn't care what the risks were; I wanted to be able

to read the Bible.

Christianity is complicated in Colombia. Although Christians are sometimes persecuted, Christianity is not illegal. It is a risk to be a Christian in public. I do not take anything for granted, but I so desperately wanted to be able to read the Bible.

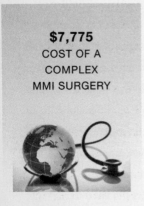

$7,775
COST OF A
COMPLEX
MMI SURGERY

All my life I had heard the Bible stories, and I knew that I loved Jesus, but I had never read the Bible. For years I prayed for God to grant me vision so I could read His Word myself. I know God answers prayers, but I did not know why He was not answering mine.

I wasn't blind, but my eyesight was poor and I had no way to get glasses. I couldn't do simple tasks like sweeping the dirt floor or cooking meals. I couldn't even have my own garden because I could not tell the weeds from the plants. It was a daylong project just to clean my small two-roomed hut.

As I grew older, my vision became worse and worse and my small radio became one of my most prized possessions. One day when I was listening, I heard that there was a Medical Ministry International eye clinic not more than a day away from where I was!

I had heard about MMI before and knew they were very smart and helped people that the doctors in Colombia could not. For the first time, I had real hope and I trusted that they would help me see.

The hardest part was the journey. After hours of riding in the open bus over the bumpy ground, my face was covered with dust. As I stood to get off the bus, I was helped down the stairs. I was so nervous, but excited at the same time. Would MMI be able to help me? Would I be able to see well enough to read?

Inside the building, I signed in and waited to meet with a nice doctor. After some tests on machines I had never seen before, the doctor came in with a pair of glasses. My hands shook as I brought them to my eyes. Blinking twice, the kind face of the doctor came into focus.

I could see! MMI had been my answer to prayer!

It has been one year since I received glasses, and now I am teaching the Bible to my friends at my house. God was so faithful to me that I had to tell others, and they believed because of it. MMI helped more than just me when they gave me my glasses; they helped everyone who comes to my house to hear about God.

María's village has been so changed by her story

and our work. The MMI team in Colombia has heeded the words of John 15:11-12, "I have told you this so that my joy may be in you and that your joy may be complete. My command is this: Love each other as I have loved you."

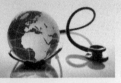

70%
OF ALL HEALTHCARE FOR THE AMAZON REGION IS PROVIDED BY MMI

Expressing our love for the Lord and His people is central to everything we do. An MMI team in San Juan, Colombia recently prayed over their patients and the village leaders, asking God to continue to help them grow and to strengthen their faith.

When the prayer was over, the opportunity was given to the Colombian people to raise their hands and come forward to receive the Gospel. The entire leadership team of the village and nearly all of the members came forward, a miracle that will last for all eternity, as the Bible says:

"For God so loved the world that he gave his one and only Son, that whoever believes in him shall not perish but have eternal life."

John 3:16

LIN TELLS A VILLAGE

In the Old Testament, Jonah had a small problem: God wanted him to go somewhere he didn't want to go.

We read, "But Jonah ran away from the Lord and headed for Tarshish" (Jonah 1:3). Of course I have no way of knowing this, but I have to wonder if he had ignored God before.

I know I have. I have felt the pull of the Lord towards something I didn't want to do, and talked myself right out of doing it. No lightning bolt came down from heaven; no booming voice shamed me from above, but looking back, I am sure I've missed a blessing or two by not following His leading.

But Jonah was—and is—God's poster boy for what happens when you don't do what He tells you. One minute Jonah was traveling merrily by boat in the opposite way God directed him, and the next thing he knew, the boat was in a storm so violent that everyone onboard feared for his life. Jonah's small problem had just gotten bigger!

You know the rest of the story: he was tossed out into the angry sea, swallowed by a giant fish, and survived for three days inside the fish's stomach. I'll bet as Jonah sat on that nasty tongue in the dark, he wished he had dealt with his problem when it was small.

Life is like that in the villages around T'Boili, Philippines. There are no doctors or nurses within a day's walk, so small medical problems become big ones. This is what happened to Lin, a gentle lady who watched as her problem grew terrifyingly huge right before her eyes:

I am an old lady of 58 and I have always worked hard in the rice fields. I have six children and have been through many rough seasons in my life. But somehow I always managed to be a help to my family, until my stomach began to grow.

At first I thought it was old age. I have always been thin, weighing less than 100 pounds, so when my stomach started to grow I was not concerned. Even though I didn't like the way it looked, I was not worried.

But it kept growing. It had been many years since my last baby, and I knew very well the signs of pregnancy; this was no baby. My husband made a few comments, trying to make me laugh, but it was starting to cause problems. My clothes didn't fit. Soon it was hard to stand up because my ankles and feet were swelling—and this was only after a few weeks.

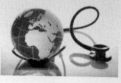

2,967
PATIENTS
SERVED IN THE
PHILIPPINES
IN 2012

My body ached from exhaustion. I could not work; all I could do was eat a little and lie back on my mat and sleep. My children tried to get me to walk, to move, but I couldn't.

I knew I should see a doctor, but that would mean traveling by foot for days and spending money we did not have. How could I do that? The few dollars my husband made a week had to first feed our youngest children, and then him and me; we barely had enough.

For two years I suffered as my stomach grew larger than it had been with any of my pregnancies. I cried at night when no one could hear me. What was wrong with me? I could barely walk; I could not make myself go to the river to wash. I wanted to die; I thought I would die.

My family was worried for me; I could see it on their faces every time they looked at me. It just made me feel worse. They had too much to worry about without worrying about me, too.

And then someone in my village told my husband about Medical Ministry International. He came to my side with the great news. The MMI clinic was not far away. It would be a long walk, but I knew I could make it; I had to.

When we arrived, we were greeted with smiling faces and kind eyes. Everyone was so helpful and supportive. After answering questions for the nurse, the doctor came in and told me there was a large tumor in my stomach and they could remove it!

The surgery was successful—but it was hard. The tumor weighed 46 pounds—half my size! I lost a lot of blood during surgery and became hypotensive—meaning my blood pressure dropped dangerously low—and hypothermic—meaning my body temperature dropped dangerously low. Losing all that blood almost cost me my life.

But the MMI team performed a miracle and word spread throughout the village about how they helped me. After hearing I was in the clinic, my village took care of my family while I recovered.

After the surgery, I only had one question: why did these strangers come to help me? I could not pay them. I did not know them. They were not related to me. Why *did they give so much?*

The answer was Jesus. Jesus loved them so they loved me. It took many days to recover but when I did, I made sure that everyone in my village knew about Jesus!

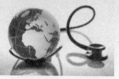

$30
AVERAGE
MONTHLY INCOME
OF AN
MMI PATIENT

Nothing is more amazing than the testimony of a life changed by the hand of God. Do you think Jonah was an effective evangelist when he finally arrived where God wanted him to go? Do you think his message was more impactful? His passion more obvious?

When we experience the miraculous power of God—and those who have chosen Christ as their Savior undoubtedly have—we have no choice but to show that love to others.

"For I have come down from heaven not to do my will
but to do the will of him who sent me.
And this is the will of him who sent me,
that I shall lose none of all those he has given me,
but raise them up at the last day."

John 6:38-39

FABIOLA'S TWO COINS

People who volunteer to do mission work or donate to a ministry do so with expectations. Whether they support the ministry with their time, their resources, or both, they want to see a return on their investment.

In ministry, this return is usually measured by the number of people who hear about Christ, how many come to salvation, or for MMI, how many volunteers we send, how many patients we see.

While these desired results are all good, they are not the only standards for success. We read in Mark 12:43-44 that Jesus doesn't count the amount of what we give, but the cost:

"Calling his disciples to him, Jesus said, 'Truly I tell you, this poor widow has put more into the treasury than all the others. They all gave out of their wealth; but she, out of her poverty, put in everything—all she had to live on.'"

Did those who had given more, like the Pharisees, consider the widow's offering a poor return on investment? Of course! But the truth is, it was all she had to give, and it was enough for Jesus. That was the whole point of the parable.

Below is the story of a woman named Fabiola from the Dominican Republic. By American standards, the gift she gave wasn't much. But it was all she had, and it spoke volumes about her gratitude.

Let her story speak to you:

These past four years have been the hardest, and I would not have been able to get through them if not for Medical Ministry International.

My husband died from HIV four years ago. Soon after, I caught pneumonia and was in a government hospital for almost a week. I had no appetite and spent most of my days just sleeping, trying my best to recover. When I was sick, I couldn't work. If I didn't work I didn't make money to buy food and with my husband gone, I was on my own.

Eventually I recovered from the pneumonia, eager to get back to work so I could begin paying my bills again. That was when the doctor told me I was HIV positive.

All he was able to offer were some prescriptions to help me fight the virus' symptoms. There was no way to completely get rid of my disease; it was something I would have for the rest of my life.

There I was, a broken widow, still trying to build my strength from the pneumonia, and I had just found out that I was HIV positive. I felt so overwhelmed, but had high expectations for the medicine. It wouldn't cure me, but I hoped it would bring a little relief.

I left the hospital with seven different prescriptions, not all of them related to the HIV, but all of them supposedly necessary. My doctor did not take the time to explain what each medication was for; he just handed me the prescriptions and I trusted him. I went home hopeful, but not happy.

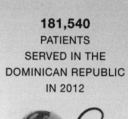

181,540
PATIENTS
SERVED IN THE
DOMINICAN REPUBLIC
IN 2012

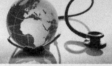

My hope did not last long. I soon realized I would not be able to get my medicine because the prescriptions could only be filled in the city and I had no money and no way to get there.

Just when I was about to give up hope, I heard about MMI. Someone in my village told me that MMI had a clinic nearby and would help me—they might even be *able to give me my medicine!*

This was the first good news I had received in a long time. The MMI clinic was much closer to my village than the city was, and I was able to make the journey in one day.

As I walked up to the fence surrounding the clinic, I began to worry. In my excitement, I had forgotten that I still had nothing to offer as payment—no money, nothing to trade for their services, not even a piece of fruit. Discouraged, I leaned against the fence, sliding my fingers through the holes of the chain link. I had come so close.

Hanging my head, I slowly began to cry. The journey had been exhausting and I hadn't eaten all day. After wiping the tears from my eyes, I looked up at the clinic one last time, wishing for a miracle.

In the distance, I saw a woman walking outside. It took me a moment to realize she was walking towards me. At first I was happy—would she invite me in? But then I had another thought. What if she was going to tell me to leave? What if she thought I was trying to cause trouble?

Just as I turned to leave, she called out to me. I didn't speak her language so I didn't know what she said, but her voice sounded kind so I knew she wasn't trying to get rid of me.

The lady introduced herself as Donna. Through broken phrases, I communicated that I wanted to be seen by a doctor, but I had no money. Donna invited me into the clinic. To be sure she knew I couldn't pay, I told her again that I had no money.

But Donna just smiled, nodded, and led me inside.

I signed in and was soon seen by a doctor, a man named Chris. While the pharmacy was preparing my medications, he told me, one by one, what each of the pills was for; it was the first time I knew what they did.

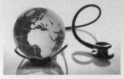

$17,179,979
VALUE OF SERVICES
PROVIDED IN THE
DOMINICAN REPUBLIC
IN US DOLLARS
LAST YEAR

I was so touched by MMI's generosity, that the people at the clinic would treat me even though I didn't have money. As I turned to leave, Donna stopped me and handed me a basket filled with clothes and soap, a beaming smile on her face. I started crying for the second time that day. This time, they were tears of joy.

I hugged Donna, said my thanks again, and left.

This past year, I went back to the MMI clinic. I wanted to see Donna and Chris and say "thank you" with two avocados, the only way I could show my *gratitude. I found Donna, gave her a big hug, and handed her my two avocados. Donna hugged me back.*

Although we still didn't understand each other's language, we were able to communicate through smiles and hugs. MMI did more than just help me with my health; they brought a smile to my face that had been missing for years.

Fabiola's story is an example of the best return of investment: she has her health and has experienced the love of God. She was so grateful to MMI that she gave all that she could—two avocados and a hug—to say "thank you."

Is that enough? It is surely enough for my God, so it is enough for me.

We cannot judge a return of investment on what we have as the recipients; we must judge it by what the giver has. Just like the widow in Mark, it is not how much you give, but how much your gift means to you.

"His master replied,
'Well done, good and faithful servant!
You have been faithful with a few things;
I will put you in charge of many things.
Come and share your master's happiness!'"

Matthew 25:21

THE GIFT OF DIDIER

We all have gifts and God wants to use all of our gifts together for His purpose. It doesn't matter if your gift is as a doctor or a stay-at-home parent, a businesswoman or a waiter; we are all gifted in some way and we all have the same calling to help the poor.

The passion of our staff is contagious and a great example of this is Erin, a physical therapist who left a comfortable life in the US to serve the people in Peru. And God has used her in more powerful ways than many doctors in that country. Her training and skill set is superior and she has re-cast children's legs after terrible past surgeries or poor leg castings. With her interventions, miracles are happening all the time. Let Erin share an example:

It's something that children in elementary school do often. With their thumb and index finger shaped in an "L" on their forehead, children often taunt weaker kids with the words, "Loser! Loser!" over and over again. No child should have to endure such bullying, but they do.

Little Didier would have been an easy target for this ridicule. His thumb and forefinger were frozen in a permanent "L." This and his other disability would have branded him for life, if not for the help we are able to provide.

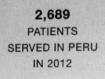

2,689
PATIENTS
SERVED IN PERU
IN 2012

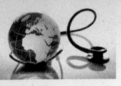

At just nine months, Didier contracted a bronchial respiratory infection. He was kept and "treated" in a local, state-run hospital. To keep him from tugging at the tubes that helped him breathe and delivered medication, the doctors and nurses pulled his right arm back over his head, overextending it, and strapped it down.

Good intentions, I am sure, but after weeks with almost no circulation, he was left with an unbending, unusable right thumb and forefinger, frozen in that taboo "L" shape.

To make matters worse, he was also diagnosed with hypotonia, a medical condition leaving him with very low muscle tone. This causes his feet to turn inward, forcing him to hyperextend his knees because his legs were too weak to hold himself.

Didier was receiving physical therapy for his hypotonia from a local hospital, and his nurses were overwhelmed by his needs. They recommended visiting Medical Ministry International's clinic to see if we could fit Didier with a leg brace to help him with the process.

I met with Didier's mother and agreed to provide her with a brace for him. When I asked if the doctors at the local hospital were doing anything for Didier's right hand, she looked confused for a moment.

She shook her head, "No." I was hardly surprised, but concerned. I knew if he didn't strengthen the muscles in his two fingers soon, chances were he would never be able to use them. We needed to work quickly.

I soon had him started on electrical muscle stimulation; it was the only way I knew to get movement back into his hand.

With a hope of improving his life, he and his mother board a bus and make the 45-minute trip twice a week to the MMI clinic. After getting off the bus, she walks another 15 minutes, carrying Didier the whole way, just to get here.

And it is worth it. Didier is now three years old and is making progress not only with walking and his two fingers, but also with cognition: he is more responsive to interaction and by the way his eyes light up, it is clear that he understands when people talk to him; before his *eyes had been dull, emotionless.*

In Peru, his disabilities would have made him an outcast. But now, with the love of a mother and the ability of MMI to meet his needs, he will have a chance at a bright future.

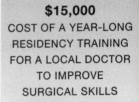

$15,000
COST OF A YEAR-LONG RESIDENCY TRAINING FOR A LOCAL DOCTOR TO IMPROVE SURGICAL SKILLS

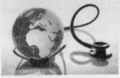

What may seem like an easy solution to us can be a miracle in other parts of the world, especially to a dedicated, loving mother like Didier's.

Now, as she sees her child being healed before her eyes, her heart is filled with gladness. And because her son is being healed, she has a heart ready and open to receive as Erin shares her faith.

> *"'But I will restore you to health*
> *and heal your wounds,' declares the Lord,*
> *'because you are called an outcast,*
> *Zion for whom no one cares.'"*
>
> ***Jeremiah 30:17***

A FRIEND LIKE CAROLINA

In Luke 5, we read a story of a bunch of normal guys who had real faith, enough faith that they knocked out the roof of a house so Jesus could heal their friend: "They went up on the roof and lowered him on his mat through the tiles into the middle of the crowd, right in front of Jesus" (19).

The faith of a friend is powerful. In the places where we work, I see firsthand some amazing acts of sacrifice and giving. These people who have nothing teach me what it is to love, to care, to be generous, to give oneself.

Carolina is one of those generous, loving people. Here she tells the story of her best friend, Luz:

I could never make it alone. I mean that. Life in our Colombian village means sharing, giving, and being there for one another.

By myself, I don't own much—a handful of rice might be the only food I have all day. Sometimes I don't have the tools I need for my garden, and I don't own a bucket to wash my clothes in.

But together with my village, I am rich. We share everything, from garden tools to water buckets and sometimes even food.

Some people in our village, like me, are too old to work anymore. My back hurts and my body is not strong like it was when I was young. I can't work long days in the fields like I used to, but I can tend the gardens in the village and wash the clothes for the men and women who work all day.

That is, I could until I got cataracts. A few years ago, my vision started getting blurry. I thought it would get better, but it just got worse—first one eye, then the other.

I was at a loss. I felt worthless and I was useless. It got so bad I couldn't tell one plant from another. I couldn't see a dog right in front of my feet. How could I help out my village if I couldn't see?

One day I sat on a stump in front of my house and cried. My friend Luz saw me at once and came to my side. She put her hand on my shoulder and encouraged me. I looked at her. Her face, a face that was as familiar to me as my own, was just a blur. I was hopeless.

But she told me people cared about me and there was still something I could do to help, to feel I had value: I could fetch the water. None of us had running water in our village; we had to carry it bucket by bucket from the river.

I had memorized the paths around my village and the walk to get water was not far. I smiled when I thought about it, the first smile in a long time. I have been carrying water for so long that my body is used to it, even though I am old.

This became my regular job, every day. Even though I would rise before the sun, it still took me most of the morning and afternoon to make the walk back and forth. I was always so tired after, but it felt good to know that I was helping everyone in my village.

Life went on until one day Luz told me something horrible, "I have cataracts, too, Carolina." Soon, she would be blind like me. I cried for her like I cried for me.

It was so sad to know what was happening to her. I knew her pain too well. Her vision worsened faster than mine and soon we were taking turns retrieving the water, switching every other day to give our aching bodies a break

543,267
LIVES
CHANGED
THROUGH MMI
IN 2012

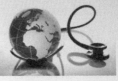

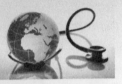

$2,000
AVERAGE
OUT-OF-POCKET
COST FOR A
VOLUNTEER
FOR ONE WEEK

and giving us each a way to contribute to the village.

I thought it would be that way until we were too sick to walk, too old to help. Then one happy summer day someone in the village told us they heard there was a Medical Ministry International clinic nearby and that the doctors could fix eyes. People just like Luz and me went there and they could see!

It was hard to sleep that night because I was so excited. After getting the water the next morning, we began our journey to the clinic. It took all afternoon to get there by bus and we had to be careful because by then, neither one of us could see much at all.

Hours later, we arrived and were welcomed by the kind doctors and nurses there. From their voices, I was sure they were good people. As they led us to our seats to wait for the sign-in, their touch was gentle, and their hands kind.

But we were just two of so many poor people who had come for help. There was only time for one of us to have the surgery; they were already full past capacity.

Luz was so kind—she let me sign up, and told me she would help me during recovery.

I agreed, but I had a plan: I would sign up and pretend that I was going to get the surgery. And then when the doctor came, I would tell him to take Luz instead. She needed the surgery more than I did.

And when the doctor came, that is exactly what I did. He was just as kind as the nurses I met earlier; he tried to convince me to have the surgery as well. He said he was sure he could make time for both of us.

But I softly explained to him, "If we both have the surgery, no one will bring the water to the village. Luz will need time to recover; she will not be able to lift heavy things for a few months. During that time, I will bring the water every day to our village."

So the doctor took a happily surprised Luz for surgery preparation. Her surgery was a success and one week later, we were making our way slowly back to the village. The doctor made me promise to come back next year if I could, and I told him I would try.

A year later, I returned with Luz. She wouldn't let me go alone because she wanted to thank me for letting her go first, and she led me the entire way there. The surgery went perfectly, and I am able to see now; we both are able to see.

Today I have a new life. I am back to tending the

gardens and washing the clothes; Luz and I make the young children get the water now. There is so much else we can do for the village and we have MMI to thank for that!

We, as the Body of Christ—like the people of Luz's village—all have our parts to play, our work, our gifts. Each part is as crucial as the other; every gift can be used for the Kingdom of God.

The same is true at Medical Ministry International. Every person who prays, who gives, who volunteers with MMI, is as much a part of the miracles as the doctors doing the surgeries. Without even one piece, our ministry is not as effective.

Do you have faith? Do something. Move in that faith and see what God will do.

"For we were all baptized by one Spirit so as to form one body—whether Jews or Gentiles, slave or free—and we were all given the one Spirit to drink. Even so the body is not made up of one part but of many."

1 Corinthians 12:13

GO OR SEND!

I had a very interesting conversation many years back with a friend of mine who is one of the world's top surgeons.

He was quite excited about how efficient our team had become, but was concerned that he did not have time to "minister" to his patients. It was not my place to say I knew the full answer, but I did share my perspective with him. Ministry is far more than just preaching; ministry is sharing—whether is it providing a glass of water or explaining what motivates you to serve—without asking for anything in return.

Every action, every word should minister to those around you. The Medical Ministry International teams use Jesus as their guide. There is no better model, but you can't just say it, you must live it.

You've read stories about our patients and learned how their lives have been changed forever because of the love and the healthcare we provide. But our patients' lives are not the only ones that are changed. Each volunteer has his or her own story, too.

The final story I will share with you is Chance's. Soon after he graduated with his nursing license from a well-known college in Mississippi, he hopped on a plane to the Amazon Region of Colombia for his second mission trip.

Please read his story, which he shared with me only days after returning to the States in June 2013:

I'll admit, I was a little worried to be going to Colombia.

I did some research about the country only after I committed to going and the more I read, the more concerned I was. Headline after headline was about the drug cartels and kidnappings; it didn't sound safe.

On top of that, there were also medical risks. While yellow fever wasn't too common, if someone did happen to get it, there was no treatment there; it was rare, but very dangerous. Everything I found was overwhelming. But I reminded myself that God was calling me to Colombia and His calming peace came over me.

I continued my pre-trip preparations: packing, praying, checking the weight of my suitcase, and repacking, followed by even more praying. And before I knew it, I was on a plane to Colombia.

We were taken from the airport to a rusty banana boat lined with wooden benches, riding low on the water. With our luggage, our team of 19 climbed onto the boat. I had to laugh, then pray, as I saw the men pile the suitcases on the back of the boat, causing it to ride even lower.

Somehow, I missed the fact that the boat ride to Santa Sofía, where we would be working for a few days, would take six hours! By the second hour, we were all sitting on life jackets and luggage, trying to get comfortable, and settling in for a great adventure.

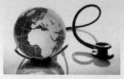

"OUR GOAL WAS JUST TO HELP WHOMEVER, ANYBODY WE COULD."

I had gone to the Dominican Republic the year before on a mission trip, but I was still surprised by what I encountered when I arrived in Colombia. The people I met were so humble and grateful even though they didn't have much. Some of the kids only owned one or two sets of clothing and lived in houses their fathers had built from whatever scraps they could find: wood, tin, tree limbs, plastic.

The people just looked happy. When I looked into their eyes, I could see their innocence. Some people think innocence is the same as naïvety, that it's a bad thing, a handicap.

But in many senses, the people in Colombia are living a better life than we are because they don't have the same distractions that we have. Being there made me realize what I truly do and don't need.

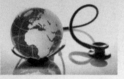

"NOT EVERYONE CAN GO ON A MISSION TRIP TO ANOTHER COUNTRY, BUT EVERYONE CAN HELP SEND SOMEONE."

During the two weeks we were there, we did everything from checking blood pressure to delousing the children. We helped out at the dentist's and at the pharmacy, too.

At the pharmacy, after we filled prescriptions, we'd sit with the patients and explain in their language what the medicine was for and why it was necessary. Many of the local doctors don't take the time to do that. Our goal was just to help whomever, anybody we could.

On our last day in Colombia, we went to a local hospital that looked like a hospital from the 1960s or 70s in the US. It was surreal to see the dated equipment. They do what they can, but even their best hospitals don't have the medical equipment that they really need.

Inside, we saw a family with a young child. I could

tell that they were very upset and our guide told us the doctors didn't know what was wrong, but they were afraid the child was dying. The child was four or five years old, and after one look I knew something was terribly wrong.

We went in, overwhelmed by our broken hearts. Putting our medical training aside, we took the child to the Healer and asked God for a miracle. We prayed, trusting, believing, asking that this child live. I've heard the stories about believers laying hands and I've read Scriptures about it, but I had never been a part of that kind of prayer before. I just had to trust that our prayers would work.

After praying, we left the hospital and soon after that, left Colombia. My two weeks there hadn't been all fun: my team and I weren't able to shower every day, we smelled sometimes and even ate bugs. I saw true poverty unlike anything I had seen before. But it was so worth it.

Just a few weeks after I returned home to Mississippi, I was on Facebook and saw an update that the child we had prayed over was healed. The doctors didn't know why, but a few days after our team left the clinic, the child recovered!

My perspective on what is truly important has changed; I have learned so much about humility, gratitude, and hospitality from the Colombian people. Those are things you'd think would be common in America. We have so much; we should be able to give so much. But oftentimes, we don't and it's amazing to see.

I know everyone can't go on a mission trip to another country, but everyone can help send someone.

Chance was able to go to Colombia and truly minister with his words and actions. His words showed the faith and love that God has for each one of His children all over the world. His actions were a testament to God's grace and compassion.

Below is the prayer Chance prayed over the child in the local hospital. There is power in prayer, and there is power in believing:

"God, I'm coming to you today. You are the ultimate Healer. I ask you, I implore You to put Your hands on this child so he can be healed and he can come to know the love that You've shown me. I pray that You would use the staff members to be Your hands and feet, that You would give them the knowledge to do their work, and that they would listen to You in their heart and save lives. Amen."

WHAT YOU CAN DO

Quite often, people ask me, "Why do you go help others when we have so much need in America?" While it is true that there are people in need right here, the needs of those we seek to serve are even more extreme. Do you remember Celia, the little girl from the Amazon who skinned her knee one day?

Well, before Medical Ministry International came, Celia might not have survived. But thankfully, we were able to help her, and today, she is back to playing, back to being a happy four-year-old. The idea that a child would die from a simple scrape seems impossible to our American minds, but it is the reality for a majority of the world.

We are blessed here in the States, and it is our responsibility to have compassion on those like Celia and her family and help them enjoy the opportunities we have been given—healthcare and basic medical necessities.

Celia is God's child, just like you and I are. She has done nothing to deserve her environment, but she cannot change it.

I am a firm believer that God challenges all believers to use the gifts He has given us, and I want to ask you: what will you give?

Before you get discouraged and think, "Sam, I'm not a doctor; I can't help," I want to encourage you—you don't have to be a doctor or a nurse to make a difference with MMI! There so many other ways to help others like Celia.

First, you can go on a project. We need dentists, surgeons, plumbers, agricultural specialists, and simply humble servants. Our teams provide care for patients under the guidance of local field staff. Each trip is short-term, usually one or two weeks, and each team builds on the work of previous teams. We serve in over 22 countries and we have more than 90 projects every year.

Second, you can pray for our ministry. Prayer is the heart of MMI. Just like Jesus was in constant communication with the Father, we believe constant prayer is the only way to do ministry. And you can pray from anywhere. Add our ministry to your morning prayer or your nightly devotional time. Pray for the patients we will see, for wisdom for our staff and volunteers, and for the countries around the world. We all need Jesus.

Third, you can support the ministry. When volunteers participate in a trip, they raise thousands of dollars to help cover costs of their travel, food, and other necessities required for them to serve. Our job is to be ready for them. We have equipment to buy and maintain, on-site staff to pay, and clinics to run in the countries we serve. Our need is great because the need for medical care is great. Every dollar you give provides $8 worth of medical care. Your gift of just $37.50 is enough to provide $300 worth of medical care!

James 2:14 reminds us all: "What good is it, my brothers and sisters, if someone claims to have faith but has no deeds? Can such faith save them?"

Please, pray and ask God to show you what you can do. Everything Jesus did, from coming to this earth as a helpless baby to dying on the cross for our sins, revolved around love and healing—spiritually and physically. Ask yourself this: what can I do to follow Jesus?

Let the healing begin with you—with your prayers, your gifts. Each of us has a role to play in caring for the orphans and the needy. Can you come? Can you pray? Can you give?

How will you help those like Celia today?

END NOTES

Copyright Page:

1. *The Holy Bible, New International Version* [Grand Rapids: Zondervan, 2011].

Dedication:

1. Shaohua Chen and Martin Ravallion, "World Bank Updates Poverty Estimates for the Developing World," Research at the World Bank. The World Bank February 17, 2010, http://web.worldbank.org/WBSITE/EXTERNAL/EXTDEC/EXT RESEARCH/0,,contentMDK:21882162~pagePK:64165401~piPK:64165026~theSitePK:469382,00.html. (accessed July 18, 2013).

Berisso Waits for God:

1. Joseph B. Verrengia, "1970-85 Famine Blamed on Pollution," Common Dreams, Associated Press July 21, 2002, http://www.commondreams.org/headlines02/0721-07.htm. (accessed July 11, 2013).
2. Ibid.
3. "Life expectancy at Birth, Total [Years]," *Data.* The World Bank, http://data.worldbank.org/indicator/SP.DYN.LE00.IN. (accessed July 11, 2013).
4. "Number of Ophthalmologists in Practice and Training Worldwide," International Council of Ophthalmology June 2012, http://www.icoph.org/ophthalmologists-worldwide.html. (accessed July 19, 2013).

God Didn't Orphan Jimmy:

1. "Orphans," *Orphans.* The United Nations Children's Fund May 25, 2012, http://www.unicef.org/media/media_45279.html. (accessed July 11, 2013).

An Answer for María:

1. "Canciller entrega reconocimient a diplomáticos como embajadores del Medio Ambiente," Naciones Unidas Oficina contra la Droga y el Delito April 23, 2008, http://wayback.archive.org/web/20080427210426/http://www.unodc.org/colombia/es/comunicado1708.html. (accessed July 11 2013).